Table of Contents

The Role of Cholesterol Levels in Life Insurance: Assessment, Implications, and Management

1. Introduction to Cholesterol and Its Significance in Life Insurance

The Impact of Cholesterol Levels on Life Insurance Applications

1. Introduction to Cholesterol and its Role in Health

There are several factors that can impact the levels of cholesterol and that can be proactively managed by a person who is applying for life insurance (especially if it is the simpler level benefit). These include diet, fat intake, nutrients (for example, folate, niacin, and B vitamins), glucose, exercise, alcohol, tobacco, thyroid function, and diabetes. In some instances, people who have contravened only one of these lifestyle factors may get an improved score if they wait 6 or 12 months. Other factors that are more difficult and costly to correct include estrogen replacement therapy, medication, and genetics, which can play a significant role in abnormal cholesterol levels (for example, familial hyperlipidemia). Cholesterol can also be known as lipid or, more colloquially, fat. Hormones are referred to as steroid synthesis. High blood cholesterol fits within the wider range of coronary artery disease risk factors, which also include smoking, diabetes, obesity, physical inactivity, hypertension, and stress. Psychologists continue to investigate the degree and manner of cholesterol links. Cholesterol has a much more limited range when it comes to morbidity and mortality, as indicated by research conducted in several other countries on mortality rates. Depending on the source, it is estimated that cholesterol may influence up to 7% of all coronary artery disease. Factors like genetics, diabetes, and race could have an effect on this statistic. The risk of complications from elevated blood cholesterol levels is as various as atherosclerosis, chest rigidity, heart attacks, angina, and other coronary artery disease states.

Cholesterol itself has no negative or positive health impact. Rather, high-density lipoprotein (HDL) cholesterol (referred to as good cholesterol), low-density lipoprotein (LDL) cholesterol (referred to as bad cholesterol), and total cholesterol/HDL ratios, among other measurements, hint at potential levels of heart disease. Values such as high HDL or low LDL, for example, are understood to be good for heart disease risk. Total cholesterol provides some indication of heart disease risk, but by itself, does not predict a high level of risk. Low HDL cholesterol is understood as a health risk. However, high total cholesterol is not necessarily a heart attack risk if it is because HDL is high. High triglycerides along with high LDL and low HDL are linked to a high heart attack risk. The level of cardiovascular risk is combined with other measurements such as blood pressure, age, and smoking status to produce a Heart Disease Risk level.

1.1. Definition and Types of Cholesterol

Cholesterol is a steroid molecule den with a single hydroxyl group or alcoholic group of a sterol, namely a steroid and alcohol compound. It is a white waxy-oily substance and derivative of steroid utilized for the body to functionalize the cell membrane and also a source of functionalizing other steroid compounds, which include the steroid (which is an essential molecule) and is used to define the formation of bile acids, adrenocortaciaol, sex hormones, as well as vitamin D. Furthermore, the term "chole" denotes bile; in alignment, it created the name of this chemical compound. Manners that radiate from the center of the LDLP, either driving the Van der Waals texture with the hydrocarbon strings with dirigenting on the water-polarizable protein surface or, mainly emphasized in this discussion, the sterolic pocket or cavity created by the hydrophobic ammonium ions and fat that is assembled for the purpose of cholesterol binding. The cholesterol is then an amphiphilic molecule structured in the unique sterical form.

The summation of cholesterol, according to ICD-9, refers to lipid metabolism. In the physics aspect, cholesterol is carried in the blood by lipoproteins. To be more exact, it is carried by some particles of high-density form, namely HDL, in addition to some particles of low-density form, LDL. The National Cholesterol Education Programme (NCEP) reported that total cholesterol levels can be categorized as "desirable" at less than 200 milligrams per deciliter (mg/dL), "borderline high" at 200-239 mg/dL, and "high" at 240 mg/dL or higher. High-density lipoprotein (HDL) particles are routinely defined as particles that contain Apolipoprotein A1, and cholesteryl ester-rich low-density lipoprotein (LDL) is designed to transport the cholesteryl esters into the peripheral tissues where, exclusive of macrophages, the effort expands an increase in the efflux of cholesterol. The cholesterols are synthesized in the liver from Acetyl coenzyme A (CoA). The liver is a significant organ where 80% of the circulating cholesterols are synthesized and designed to be transported in the blood. Additionally, the cholesterols are carried in the blood by lipoproteins, which then allow the cholesterols to reach the surface of the cell.

1.2. Functions of Cholesterol in the Body

In addition, within the plasma, cholesterol is the substrate for steroidogenesis, which is the process through which the tissues specifically produce steroid hormones such as progesterone, glucocorticoids, androgens, estrogens, and Vitamin D. Overall, cholesterol affects the development of the fetal brain and a woman's ability to breastfeed, our ability to process food, our ability to protect ourselves against infectious diseases, to initiate tissue repair, to protect neural synapse, to transmit signals along neurons, to innovate strategies to obtain evolutionary advantage, to control the degrees of freedom of transmembrane proteins, to distinguish sperm cells, eggs, and the tissues that generate them, female characteristics, and male characteristics.

For instance, cholesterol is a fundamental component of cellular membranes. It also helps modulate the fluidity of these cellular structures, which is critical for organisms to be able to proliferate and for tissues to become differentiated. Because cholesterol is selectively distributed within the plasma membranes of a human neuron or an antigen-presenting macrophage, this distribution helps in the conformation of the proteins which are responsible for the transmission of signals within. The ability of cholesterol to form lipid rafts is also vital in maintaining the rigid submembrane cytoskeletal spectrin-actin network, providing lateral movement of plasma membrane proteins, including mobile surface receptors and cell-cell adhesion molecules.

Cholesterol has been wrongly implicated in the development of cardiovascular problems. It is essential to mammals in the same way that every person has a unique biological individuality. This is basically because cholesterol is present in almost all cells in the body, playing specific functions in each of them.

2. Significance of Cholesterol Levels in Life Insurance

Producers are aware of the significance of high cholesterol levels primarily because of the increased costs associated with a higher death rate from coronary artery disease (CAD). As a result, individuals with high cholesterol levels must pay higher mortality and morbidity underwriting charges to receive life insurance coverage. The premium that prospective policyholders with undesirable cholesterol levels will pay are substandard rates. If an insured person is not insurable, there are no policyholders, agents, or insurers. Therefore, it is logical that this divergence in bias results from a difference in observed mortality. High rates must be charged if statistically high hazard rates exist.

According to the Centers for Disease Control and Prevention, cholesterol levels are a hot topic in the United States. In the last few years, professionals have begun discussing current statistics revealing the relationship of cholesterol levels with heightened risks of heart disease within both men and women. High blood cholesterol is a condition in which the cholesterol level in the blood is higher than normal. The Centers for Disease Control and Prevention report that 7 percent of children born in the United States in 1981 had high cholesterol levels. To address these high figures, the National Cholesterol Education Program and the National Institutes of Health launched an all-encompassing medical research and information campaign becoming one of the most successful campaigns ever. In a very short time, every professional, from laymen to medical experts, had been exposed to the news that keeping cholesterol levels down could help protect those at risk from cardiac incidents. Authorities recommended a total of four major lifestyle changes in diet and exercise.

2.1. Why Life Insurance Companies Consider Cholesterol Levels

Even when offered a life insurance policy, some seeking a policy may suffer from a phenomenon known as application inertia. This refers to a condition where people either don't bother or don't want to face the whole process of applying for life insurance coverage. Unfortunately, this can have serious financial consequences for the loved ones as, traditionally, funeral expenses and likely other death-related costs are settled from the benefits of life insurance. Usually, these expenses are paid first, even before a will is read and other funding can be documented. Aside from application inertia as a reason for either no coverage, unaffordable coverage or a rejected application, the underwriting process is laborious enough that it can serve as a disincentive to apply for life insurance. However, the answer would not be to forego the purchase just because of the relative price; instead, like any other important purchase, consumers are urged to strive to find a cost-effective plan from a financially stable company.

Risks associated with elevated cholesterol, such as an increased likelihood of having a heart attack or stroke, have led life insurance carriers to take cholesterol levels very seriously when determining whether to issue a policy. Generally, the higher the cholesterol level(s), the higher the rates charged by the carriers. However, if the rates are too high, the insurance may be unaffordable, and individuals may skip having the coverage altogether. That is why, when cholesterol levels are elevated, it is a good idea to work with an independent agent who has access to many different carriers. While it may be possible for some individuals working with an agent with knowledge of the underwriting and product options for rates to qualify for some level of coverage, often at a better price, it is important to research the options available not only from the premiums charged but also from an important factor to consider: the financial ratings of the company.

2.2. How Cholesterol Levels Affect Premiums

Insurers may choose to make use of this by including cholesterol clauses in contracts. The existence of such clauses is cited as a reason for collecting medical information in the life insurance industry. Specifically, a cholesterol clause allows insurers to offer applicants a policy with a higher risk loading if they are diagnosed with high cholesterol and to offer a lower risk loading if applicants are screened and can demonstrate that their cholesterol is below a certain level.

High cholesterol levels are one measure used by insurers to assess risk and are indicative of long-term health. High levels of cholesterol have been shown to increase the risk of circulatory disease in the long term. Hypothetically, insured individuals with high cholesterol levels at the time of application present a higher risk in the future and should therefore be charged more expensive premiums. Whether firms are currently underpricing the risk associated with high cholesterol is unknown, but there is some evidence that monetary incentives can encourage individuals to control their cholesterol levels.

Once underwriters have ascertained the risk level of potential applicants, they will group them into classes of insured persons with similar risk profiles. The purpose is to allocate premium according to the risk of each class. The class system will inevitably result in a degree of adverse selection. Smokers who apply for insurance are not representative of all smokers, i.e. high-risk smokers may be more likely to apply.

Life insurance companies assess applicants using a range of criteria to determine the risk they must assume and consequently what premium they should be charged. Risk factors typically include the applicant's age, sex, smoking status, and state of health. Typically, those in good health will be charged a standard premium, while those with greater health risks or poorer medical history will be charged higher premiums according to the sought of financial exposure the insurer would face if the applicant was to die. If there is a sufficient increase in risk, underwriters may decline the application.

3. Factors Affecting Cholesterol Levels

Dieting, blood volume, endogenous alcohol levels, and bird flu can affect cholesterol levels. Due to hormonal aspects such as the reproductive life period, cholesterol levels of women differ from those of men, who raise more issues than men. Due to fluctuations, the menstrual phase also plays a role. Many studies, however, have failed to show the direct relationship between hormones and adverse events, including the lack of an increased risk of CHD in postmenopausal but hormone-replaced women. The fact that birth control pills contain a relatively low amount of estrogens and progesterone could well be the reason for the smaller increase in cholesterol levels than in pregnant women. Cholesterogenesis does get accelerated with pregnancy and, during pregnancy or shortly after delivery, the TAT enzyme does not affect clot breakdown. In addition, complying with, for a short period, serious illnesses or severe physical ailments is compatible with low cholesterol levels. Animals that became sickly through specially formulated diets, conversely, may be rapidly rejuvenated. Cholesterol levels may therefore indirectly indicate a person's overall health status. Symptoms of these problems are, of course, often evident and increase the likelihood of the blood test being censored. Note exists of exposure, fatalities, major surgery, blood loss, burns, hyperthermia, or hypothermia, the use of radiation, and poisoning of pesticides. It is also known that EMG and CPK levels lower lipid levels in muscle enzyme ratio.

Several factors affect cholesterol levels. Occasionally, diabetic status may be overlooked. It is well documented that in type II diabetes mellitus, HDL-C is lowered. Some non-diabetics have a high fasting insulin level, which interestingly is thought to be related to insulin resistance. This is particularly true for South African and other dark-skinned population groups, who are relatively more prone to developing CHD at an early age. Although high total cholesterol and LDL-C levels do increase in South Africans as they approach their fifties, the levels are very seldom as low as those of their counterparts in other countries. Their higher levels throughout life would also support the use of some South African risk tables, which predict higher levels. Additionally, a number of reports indicate that cholesterol levels may be increased within a week or two of a patient contracting infections, also supporting the belief that a raised immune response may be incompatible with low cholesterol levels.

3.1. Genetics and Family History

Since the time of insurance company share issues in the mid to late 1990s, there have been significant developments in the genetics of atherosclerotic diseases and the relationship between LDL cholesterol levels and atherosclerotic diseases. Some 40-60% of the total variance in plasma levels of LDL cholesterol is genetically determined, and somatic cell genetics and molecular genetic studies have identified more than 50 polymorphic genes, all of which are associated with variations in LDL cholesterol levels. Despite considerable effort, more than 90% of the genetic contribution to interindividual variation in levels of LDL cholesterol remains to be discovered. Furthermore, a number of additional genes, none of which have been implicated in the etiology of raised levels of LDL cholesterol, have been shown to have a potential epigenetic influence on coronary artery disease during the first year of life. A prevalence ratio of 150 may lead to 3,000 cases/year of hypercholesterolemia.

The use of paneling hypothetical lives

3.2. Diet and Lifestyle Choices

Diet and lifestyle can have a significant if not immediate impact on high cholesterol levels. According to the study, it can take as little as seven days for irresponsible dietary choices to adversely affect one's health, if not affect one's cholesterol levels. After just one week on a high-fat, high-cholesterol diet, serum cholesterol levels average about 5% higher than they were before the diet began. Differences by gender included a 7%-12% increase for women and a 4%-7% increase for men. At the food level, individuals who consumed meals with butter saw their cholesterol levels increase by 5%. By contrast, the individuals who had margarine experienced a 5.5% increase in cholesterol levels.

As a rule, how well people address conditions associated with high cholesterol levels is a variable that can be easily measured, observed, and potentially improved. Since high cholesterol levels often stem from diet and lifestyle, diet and lifestyle choices are clear factors in play. In fact, many life insurance applications ask detailed questions regarding what one eats, how an individual's weight has fluctuated, or whether an applicant is a smoker. Why do these things matter? Obese applicants or those with a high-fat diet tend to display such choices in their cholesterol levels. Based on their answers to such questions, individuals can gauge how much, if any, additional cholesterol they might be generating and their general and regional health is likely improving also.

3.3. Medical Conditions and Medications

The risk class of the facing healthy or unhealthy applicants that suffer from chronic conditions is different for healthy or unhealthy applicants applying for life insurance protection. The motivation for this paper is to compare the increase in the risk class rating for medical information against the increase in the rating from treated and non-treated high blood pressure and high cholesterol values when they are the only known information. The further results based on the last large company update demonstrate that underwriting models which use easily available medical condition information are chargeable to capitalize on between 55% and 95% of this information. This highlights the importance of the history of any of the build conditions in predicting the long-term mortality risk for underwriters. It also indicates the additional information a complete and thorough investigation report can contain.

In the industry, we have the medical conditions called formally as build. Some of the common medical conditions that are collected are cancer, diabetes, heart or heart-related conditions, mental or nervous conditions, musculoskeletal and bone conditions, pregnancy, substance or alcohol abuse, disorders of the blood, high blood pressure, and high cholesterol.

It is not concerning for consumers to know various Medicare supplement plans. More so, understanding the difference between Plan F vs G helps the consumers make an informed decision. They can then select the suitable supplement plans that align with their requirements. However, with a lifestyle that involves a lot of unhealthy food, genetics that predispose them to genetic conditions, and a fast-paced life with less time to do physical activity, there has been a rise in the number of health conditions. The treatment of these conditions is also varied and involves lifestyle changes and medication.

4. Measuring Cholesterol Levels

These will highlight the role of hormones which will, as doctors treat existing health conditions, become much like the ultimate pacemaker as well as cardioactive metabolites. Cholesterol will be found to be the control metabolite to land levels in both heart patients and their cardiac regulation transmitters. Furthermore, that serum in relationship to land levels is the best housekeeping guide to prevent both future and not so random funerals. As the number of heart attacks approaches tension table values, so will those applicants who know their mortality assessment, and blood serum cholesterol, be eligible for reduced premium life policies.

Mortality prediction numbers, considered by the Society of Actuaries and most underwriters, raise the issue of "100" integers versus values meeting regression analysis needs. Mortality integers (1) from best to (10) showing the greatest history of mortality are based initially upon blood serum. However, to predict current health and identify those individuals with potential or existing health conditions that are made evident by elevated blood serum cholesterol will require much finer separation. Just as medical science has moved from extracting bodily humours from their unique control centers, mankind is now at the threshold of recognizing single point control centers for most bodily processes.

4.1. Cholesterol Testing Methods

We clarify the agreements and differences between test methods, highlight how difficult pre-analytical and analytical issues may impact overall health assessment. To test for cholesterol levels, there are several traditional and nonconventional cholesterol level tests. Historically, traditional tests include prediction methods based on observable non-cholesterol tests. Newer methods include an atherosclerotic cardiovascular disease (ASCVD) risk score to guide cholesterol-lowering treatment levels. Despite the high volume of cholesterol tests, these are likely to be far from optimal. Guidelines for cholesterol and cholesterol levels are updated when new evidence becomes available. Recommendations on what cholesterol levels are considered optimal or non-optimal may change due to technological advancements.

Determining how cholesterol pathways are altered in the disease state to enable cholesterol testing with greater predictive power is challenging based solely on analysis of specific cholesterol-related biomarkers in serum collected during wellness and disease testing. New technologies promise to increase the molecular types of analytes or sensitivity to low-abundance molecular changes that may increase the predictive power (or earlier detection) which result in cholesterol level elevation. New technologies could improve the process by which non-traditional cholesterol-related biomarkers are determined and incorporated into cholesterol tests. In the next section, we describe how the current methods for measuring cholesterol and cholesterol blood levels from medical exam blood and serum samples.

4.2. Interpreting Cholesterol Test Results

Low-density lipoprotein (LDL) cholesterol is the key culprit in heart disease, and levels should be minimized. Guidelines suggest that your healthy LDL cholesterol level should depend on your individual cardiovascular risk profile. For example, someone with a 10% 10-year absolute risk (the percentage chance of having a heart attack or stroke in the next 10 years) can aim for a lower level than someone with a 5% 10-year risk. The following list is a guide as to what the optimal range is depending on your risk.

To allow underwriters to accurately assess risk, the results of the cholesterol test must be interpreted properly within the age and sex of the applicant. Each life insurance company will have its own specific reference range as to what it considers normal, but health practitioners place considerable reliance on national guidelines when assessing risk based on the results. It is important to remember that some laboratory references will contain only absolute figures while many references will include desirable ranges. The following section is concerned with the topics of low-density lipoprotein, high-density lipoprotein, and cholesterol.

5. Understanding the Relationship Between Cholesterol and Health

LDL particles are responsible for depositing cholesterol in tissues and are often referred to as the "bad cholesterol." High levels of LDL-C, particularly increased small, dense LDL particles, are associated with an increased risk of cardiovascular events. HDL particles are responsible for picking up cholesterol and returning it to the liver where it is removed from the body and is therefore often referred to as the "good cholesterol". High levels of HDL-C provide cardiovascular protection. Finally, VLDL particles are made by the liver and transport triglycerides to tissues. After removal of triglycerides, VLDL turns into LDL. High levels of VLDL-C are also associated with an increased risk of cardiovascular issues. High levels of small, dense LDL particles (particles that transport cholesterol and triglycerides) together with low HDL and high triglyceride levels are associated with the metabolic syndrome, a type of pre-diabetes that increases the risk of coronary and vascular disease (CVD).

Cholesterol is found in every cell of the body and serves important functions, including the production of sex and stress hormones, bile production (needed for digestion), and the synthesis of Vitamin D, which is important for bone health and the immune system. Cholesterol is synthesized in the liver and has complex interactions with what we eat. Diet quality and the amount of cholesterol in foods impact the amount of cholesterol produced by the liver and, in turn, cholesterol in the bloodstream. Cholesterol is transported in the body by lipoproteins. There are several types of lipoproteins, but the most important in assessing cardiovascular health are High Density Lipoproteins (HDL), Low Density Lipoprotein (LDL), and Very Low-Density Lipoprotein (VLDL).

5.1. Health Risks Associated with High Cholesterol

High levels of bad cholesterol can result in fatty deposits building up in blood vessels and clogging arteries. This combination of high cholesterol and heart disease is a major health threat. High cholesterol levels can have a serious influence on the likelihood of having a heart attack or a stroke, which are both considered life-threatening. High cholesterol usually has no signs or symptoms and can be detected only by means of a blood test. The high-risk groups for cardiovascular diseases are men older than 55, women older than 65, anyone with established cardiovascular disease, and people with hyperlipidemia. As part of a healthy lifestyle, a well-balanced diet is very important to maintain appropriate levels of good cholesterol because it helps protect against heart disease. Factors that influence cholesterol levels are age, gender, genetics, obesity, and diet.

The impact of cholesterol levels is a very important health factor in the assessment of an application, and for that reason, a detailed explanation of this factor is provided here. Cholesterol is a fatty substance called a lipoprotein and is carried around the bloodstream in packages of proteins. Two types of packages exist, one called low density and the other high-density lipoprotein. The high-density lipoprotein is known as good cholesterol, and the low density is referred to as bad cholesterol. The body needs cholesterol to function properly, and if cholesterol levels are too low, it can be as harmful as if cholesterol levels are too high.

5.2. Benefits of Maintaining Healthy Cholesterol Levels

There are many substances in the diet that are difficult, or indeed, impossible to convert into energy by the body. Certain vitamins, such as A, D, E, and K are found only in the presence of cholesterol, in foods of animal origin, in the form of fats and oils, and other lipids. Much of the cholesterol obtained from the diet by the human being is eventually lost into the intestinal tract because most of it is not absorbed into the blood. Animal observations on dogs have demonstrated that the pulvinar of the small intestine plays an important role in the regulation of cholesterol absorption. Although much dietary cholesterol is lost through the intestinal tract, we would eventually expect any situation in which the body becomes the second chockfull of cholesterol. Such a body might be able to consume the normal amount of fuel so that, when the balance can no longer be achieved, the blood may become loaded with cholesterol.

The term heart disease has been used to describe the end result of several physiological changes that can occur in the organ known as the heart. The real purpose of the heart as a muscle is to act as a pump that continuously supplies a large amount of blood, and therefore oxygen, to the body at all times. Some series of experiments carried out show that an organ, such as the heart, with these characteristics, would have to consume large amounts of fuel, especially if we consider that no rest period is built into the activity of the heart. Four hundred and twenty-five metric tons of blood are pumped continuously through the vessels of the heart as weight increases and decreases, as determined by the needs of the other body tissues. Animal observations support the view that the physiological condition of the body tissues plays a major controlling role in the beating activities of the heart. Animal evidence also shows the presence of mechanisms in the body to compensate for relatively small errors that might develop in the control of these consuming activities. For the body to maintain its normal routines, however, the supply of fuel must always equal its demand.

For the person currently not concerned with their cholesterol level, or even for a person who has recently been told that their cholesterol is too high, it is difficult, or nearly impossible, to appreciate the medical problems that can come about as a result of uncontrolled high cholesterol levels. Anyone, especially people who are fortunate enough to apparently enjoy perfect health, who are advised, because of high cholesterol levels, to adopt strict dietary or medical treatment, at considerable expense, would naturally tend to meet that advice with some reserve, and would expect to be told, in detail, what the benefits of such strict diets or other treatment might be. The simple facts are that people have died as a direct result of high, and in some instances, extraordinarily high cholesterol levels; those who have died were as healthy and as conscious as you and I are at present. In most of these instances the mechanism of death was due to heart disease, and, specifically, myocardial infarction.

6. Strategies for Improving Cholesterol Levels

Medication is always what someone will fall back on if cholesterol levels just refuse to go down. The size and consistency of our cholesterol levels will change and you will feel much better on a day in and day out basis. There is no such thing as instant gratification in attempts to change our cholesterol levels. It is very possible that you will be more motivated to take control of our nutrition and fitness rather than just relying on immediate medication if this were not the case, as medication is a way out that is not necessarily permanent. If you do try to achieve immediate gratification, then reduce fast food totally so that our cholesterol levels will reduce somewhat to get you a little bit more motivated. However, reducing fast food totally for some people may be an unrealistic goal to have, dependent on what drives you emotionally.

Cholesterol levels can often seem like an obscure piece of our puzzle to health, but the truth is that we have a good idea of what causes cholesterol levels to become elevated. To lower cholesterol levels, take charge of your nutrition, your physical fitness, your sleep, and even your ideas. It is possible for someone to actually be overweight yet not have the high cholesterol that usually accompanies obesity. Regular physical fitness, in which the heart rate is kept high for sustained periods of time, has been linked to reducing bad cholesterol levels. Instead, you should chart our cholesterol levels and eating habits, specifically any foods that trigger overeating, so that you can alter your eating habits accordingly.

6.1. Healthy Diet and Nutrition Tips

There are usually no symptoms to warn you if you have high blood cholesterol. A simple blood test can determine your cholesterol level. The test is painless and can help save your life! Children age 2 and above should have their cholesterol tested if their parents or grandparents developed heart disease before age 55 for men or before age 65 for women, or they have other risk factors such as obesity, diabetes, or high blood pressure.

2. Know your cholesterol level.

Watch your total and saturated fat intake. Choose foods with unsaturated fats (such as olive, peanut, or canola oil). Consume more fish - high in omega-3 fatty acids - at least two times per week (2-3 grams/day may reduce triglyceride levels). Eat more fruits, vegetables, bread, and cereal. Eat less meat, whole milk, cream, and foods with coconut or palm oil. Avoid foods with partially hydrogenated oils. Avoid foods high in cholesterol. Eat 20-30 grams of dietary fiber per day (10-25 grams of the edible fiber) from a variety of sources. Limit caloric intake to balance caloric needs with caloric intake to help maintain desirable body weight. Keep alcohol intake moderate. Keep protein intake moderate.

Optimizing a healthy diet reduces your body's demand for cholesterol. Below are some nutritional guidelines suggested by the American Heart Association.

6.2. Physical Activity and Exercise Recommendations

Most people are not at risk of developing any problems by engaging in low-level activities. Low-level activities such as gardening, housework, and short walks frequently can be beneficial. People normally decide to start an exercise program for reasons that are based more on emotion than sound thinking. Perhaps they need to lose weight or decrease their blood cholesterol. It could also be that a gym has opened nearby. People need to think carefully about their exercise program rather than just jumping right in. Because habits are often hard to break and harder to change, an incorrect or inappropriate exercise program can be hard to stop. When people start out with an exercise program that is difficult to continue, they risk exercising too hard and risking injury and increased stress. On the other hand, the ideal exercises for a person to execute are the ones that are easy to continue. When individuals do exercises correctly, perform them on a daily basis, and set realistic goals, they will benefit most from their exercise program. When injured, individuals should resist taking time off from the forced inactivity caused by the injury if at all possible. In many instances, other forms of exercise are available. When it is essential to take time off, one will still wish to continue as many enjoyable activities as possible.

The relationship between physical activity and health is well established. Physical activity releases endorphins and helps to manage stress. Additionally, it helps to control calories and reduce undesirable levels of plasma cholesterol, blood pressure, and glucose. While an individual's health is an important factor in any life insurance purchase, individuals also need to consider the health of their finances. Any comprehensive set of guidelines for physical activity should try to contribute to the maintenance of the individual's health and the reduction of employers' healthcare costs. The recommendations of the Center for Disease Control are a valuable resource for any individual and can also be implemented as corporate wellness programs.

7. Cholesterol Management and Life Insurance Applications

Current assessment practices for cholesterol levels lie in question both from an initial (either for employment or life insurance) standpoint as well as from an insurable perspective. Undoubtedly, steps toward the development of improved cholesterol assessment practices could play a prominent role in contributing to increased consumer awareness as well as to future applications. Indeed, current blood cholesterol level discrimination found in life insurance applications may detract from the dominant objective to serve applicants competitive levels of products desired by an economic risk discrimination criterion.

In the wake of these statistics and the associated medical advancements, life insurance underwriting has adopted guidelines for assessing an applicant's risk based on a variety of factors that include blood pressure as well as blood cholesterol levels. At least these guidelines have been established for individuals not applying for wasting disease, applicants over age 65, and coverages in excess of $500,000. Recent attempts have been made to increase the awareness of government programs to control cholesterol levels of the general public. Without these efforts, steps geared to increase cholesterol management in a life insurance setting will surely fail.

7.1. Steps to Take Before Applying for Life Insurance

Since the basic product function of a life insurance policy is to pay a certain sum of money on the death of the insured person, most people are best served by buying term insurance which provides the most coverage for the dollar. You will need different amounts of insurance at various times. Chances are, however, there will be a point at which it makes more sense to convert some of the old term insurance to a more permanent form of insurance. In that case, a variety of ways will be available to cover the remaining needs more permanently while still providing for increased needs in the future.

What kind of policy should I buy?

The ideal time to apply for life insurance is during your peak earning years. The group with the most need for insurance is made up of young marrieds with children. For those just starting out, many competing demands on income mean that hard choices are necessary. Appropriately priced, life insurance can provide the necessary protection. While smaller amounts of insurance will be needed when current earnings are at lower levels, everyone will have short-term needs for insurance at different times of life. Think about buying larger policies at younger ages. It means converting the coverages to smaller and less expensive policies after the need has declined.

When should I apply for life insurance?

There are several questions to answer or issues to resolve before applying for life insurance. Life insurance is a contract between two parties, the policyholder and the insurance company. In return for paying money to the insurance company, the policyholder expects the company to pay a predetermined sum of money to a predetermined beneficiary when the policyholder dies. The main function of life insurance is to provide income to the beneficiaries of policyholders after their deaths.

7.2. How to Improve Cholesterol Levels for Better Insurance Rates

You will also need to quit smoking for obvious reasons. Most importantly you should talk to your abs. So the first way to improve your cholesterol levels is to eat a heart-healthy diet. Nutritional experts strongly recommend a diet that is rich in whole grains, fruits, and vegetables, and that is low in unhealthy fats, cholesterol, and sodium. Soluble fiber, which can help reduce bad cholesterol levels, is found in oats, apples, oranges, and pears, for example. Once again, you should stop dieting and start with better nutrition for the rest of your life. Start with a dietitian and then read more about appropriate substitutions. By this time, you may already be doing some of these things every day. If you are not, then make it a priority to really try to follow the instructions every day. After months of following these guidelines, you can return to your insurance agent for another test or checkup to see if your payment plan can be adjusted. Keep in mind that rates can only be adjusted at the end of a term or when you buy a policy with a better rating - the carriers can never raise the cost of a policy based on medical screenings.

First of all, and this is a little silly, you should increase your intake of soluble fiber. You can find it in apples, barley, beans, oats, and oranges. Research shows that eating just a half-cup a day of many of these foods can lower cholesterol by 10 percent within a month. Moving on from diet and nutrition, losing at least a little spare tire can help to lower cholesterol levels. Even losing just 5 to 10 pounds can have a positive impact. You should try to exercise for a minimum of 30 minutes, five times a week. Moderate exercise, such as taking a brisk walk, is best. A little bit of alcohol per day can be good for your heart but keep it to no more than a drink of alcohol per day for women and those over 65 and no more than two drinks per day for men under 65.

8. Case Studies and Real-Life Examples

This intelligent underwriting solution will help this application process be corrected, be efficient, and the underwriting decision can be made with more confidence. In short, using intelligent underwriting or medical underwriting principles, which selectively targets applicants, can assist the life insurance companies to identify genuine applications seeking coverage that has genuine needs at the best acceptable terms. With the intelligent process, life insurance companies can better distinguish between those who make inaccurate representations, who are conflicted about their desire for coverage, while motivating the customers to improve both their corporeal and financial health.

In the above cases, Mr. A and Mr. B or his agent can make inaccurate representations when applying for a life insurance policy to avoid facing additional chargeable premiums or difficulties in the underwriting process, which may affect the success of the life insurance application. In the event that these cases are purely business sourcing errors, and no additional underwriting requirements are generated to capture the actual health and financial risks of the life insurance company, the life insurance companies are losing out in both premium and earnings, potentially leaving dangerous gaps in protection for the parties concerned.

Case study 2: Mr. B is a 45-year-old pharmacist applying for a life insurance income replacement coverage (5 times annual income) for 5 years. Without assuming that he has high cholesterol, his application will be the standard underwriting required. Should Mr. B be discovered to have high cholesterol, his application will also face an additional chargeable premium if he fails underwriting required.

Case study 1: Mr. A is a 35-year-old banker applying for a life insurance protection coverage of 10 times annual income for a 20-year period. Without assuming that he has high cholesterol, his application will be the standard underwriting required. Should Mr. A be discovered to have high cholesterol, his application will face an additional chargeable premium, coverage may be loaded, or underwriting may be postponed to a new underwriting limit.

Due to data privacy, we are unable to obtain real-life examples to share here. However, we are able to provide case studies of applicants who face difficulties in their application due to high cholesterol.

8.1. Impact of Cholesterol Levels on Insurance Coverage Decisions

A traditional solution from financial theory to this problem is that applicants should be compelled to submit to some "medical testing." This raises the question: In what manner, if any, are cholesterol levels measured relevant to insurance coverage decision making? Also, is the cholesterol measurement the first or only test underwritten by a prospective policyholder by the insurance company willing to assume certain health risks? Finally, it is also worth considering potential concerns for the insurers about adverse selection. Profitable business for insurance companies, on the other hand, would be lost if a large proportion of the sales were drawn from poor health risks classified as standard rates.

The request for life insurance coverage is introduced first. Many insurance companies regard cholesterol as an essential tool for assessing mortality risk, and as a result of the questionable reliability of other tests recently, a newfound interest in cholesterol as a predictor of future life-threatening diseases may also have affected insurance companies. The presenting agent suggests that cholesterol is currently the most important risk factor. As an example, the presentation makes a distinction among three classes of insurance coverage: ordinary, a preferred policy, universal, and a life policy product with an exceptional return on premiums, proposed in 1987 - universal plus. They argue that insurance companies' decision-making process for selecting insureds might be improved.

9. Conclusion and Future Perspectives

The discovery of a comparable visiting point, like blood testing, can assist in most individually visited marketing operations. Other than global practices like serological confirmations, are acknowledged today to evaluate information, normally blood examined lumber, the levels of cholesterol as well triglycerides, also quick to initiate. In the evaluation of insurance decisions, these specific laboratory tests could be utilized to recognize dissimilar risk levels. Providing a tailoring approach to the marketplace seldom circles and differentiated policies based on cholesterol blood tests. A direct sequence of cholesterol measures emphasizing the amount of deceit, minimum damage, or quite insignificant, which encourages, in the frame of good size, the business of the insurance company.

Life insurance marketplace is a complicated area because it is constantly engaged in progressing health technologies and necessitates dependable health, which is vital for insurance firms. There are remarkably sudden future advantages, as claims depend on far beyond the customary period. It's characteristics like this that mainly permit life insurance firms to offer many products and value boosts. Lofty standards in matter connection, skill, and assurance are generally associated with low ethics, with the application of the principles receiving increasing disapproval. On the other hand, the amount of discriminating operations, many of which authorize input from the candidate, ask for physical examination, neuro tests, or analysis and understanding of the applicant's physical health.

9.1. Summary of Key Points Discussed

The impact of cholesterol levels on the underwriting of life insurance is not specifically captured through MIB codes, nor, due to adverse selection issues with voluntary testing, is it believed to be the area of as significant concern as some other DoB codes. While cholesterol level tests exist (MIB codes 2 and 5), they may be taken by older individuals for reasons largely unrelated to life insurance. For example, some persons have voluntarily taken cholesterol tests for baseline or similar reasons in anticipation of future elective surgery or as part of health screenings sponsored by community groups.

Insurers use information about the medical histories of proposed insureds in making underwriting assessment decisions. Some DoB Medical Information Bureau (MIB) codes indicate applicants' cholesterol levels at some time in the past, if testing was performed. This study of 20 life insurers' underwriting rules involving MIB codes related to cholesterol concluded that only about half of the insurers actually used cholesterol test results. An in-depth discussion of suggested scenarios involving code 2 values and code 5 values. A primary benefit of this study is to give companies a baseline, probably not widely available elsewhere, as to what leading insurers' underwriting rules are in this area.

9.2. Emerging Trends in Cholesterol Management and Insurance Industry

9.1.3. Total Cholesterol (TC) Cut-off Values for Smoker and in Smoker Double Measurement Until 4th June, insurance applicants who need insurance except for the highest rating were advised to fast and declare that they had, as per application questions on the schedule and any other application forms in use. Total Cholesterol (TC) results for smoker and in-smoker would have resulted in 5.20, 5.60, 6.00, 6.40, 6.80, 7.20, and 7.60 mmol/L.

9.1.2. Lp(a), Lp-PLA2, Lp(a), and Lp-PLA2 tests, for which insurers had been allowed by the regulator to mark up smokers' premium rates compared with non-smokers in some fast approval territories for many years, became widespread in 2010. These functional blood tests more directly assess the risk of heart disease and stroke. Statins have no influence on Lp(a) values, but they do reduce the Lp-PLA2 level. Lp-PLA2 is reviewed as a higher level educated exclusion condition in Section 4.1.1.

September 2013. For now, the calculation of TC:HDL using the more cumbersome dual measurement style will continue until the market adapts to the new tested method without criticism of its high accuracy and reliability.

The Role of Cholesterol Levels in Life Insurance: Assessment, Implications, and Management

1. Introduction to Cholesterol and Its Significance in Life Insurance

Cholesterol is usually a small, fat-like substance made in the liver, and it is present throughout the blood. This fat is crucial due to its role in building cell membranes and essential hormones. But too much cholesterol in the blood, often from poor food choices, can be harmful. Cholesterols are transported through the bloodstream by molecules called "lipoproteins" (combinations of proteins and fat). There are five forms of lipoproteins, all of which carry varying quantities of cholesterol and triglycerides. Lipoproteins can be divided into two categories: low-density lipoprotein (LDL) and high-density lipoprotein (HDL). Research indicates that monitoring the patient's level of LDL (LDL-C) is more indicative of CAD than measuring their level of TC, and that origin is a better predictor of disease than total cholesterol. The risk of developing CAD is higher when LDL-C levels are higher. HDL cholesterol levels are associated with a lower risk of developing CAD, which protects HDL-C.

This chapter will focus on understanding the role of cholesterol levels in the domain of life insurance. A basic understanding of what cholesterol is, and what role it plays in the human body, is essential before we delve deep into the topic. The importance of cholesterol as a risk factor in the assessment and underwriting of life insurance proposals is well known. High cholesterol levels can prove to be detrimental to an individual's ability to buy life insurance. For those who have been able to effect a life insurance contract at standard terms, periodic evaluations of cholesterol levels are an important aspect of their risk management. A number of factors impinge on the choice of cholesterol level cut-offs. Whenever such cut-offs are influenced, it is good to reassess the position at regular intervals. In this chapter, cholesterol will encompass total cholesterol (TC), which is considered to be the sum of low-density lipoprotein cholesterol (LDL-C) and high-density lipoprotein cholesterol (HDL-C), plus one-fifth of the triglycerides (as underwater glycerol), if the plasma triglyceride level is high. A brief contemporary overview of serum lipids and plaque initiation has been included.

2. Establishing Acceptable Cholesterol Levels for Life Insurance Purposes

Mortality experience studies and conservative underwriting make it possible to establish cholesterol levels that make people uninsurable. Terminology often used to describe those cholesterol levels is "acceptable" and "unacceptable" criteria, and the term most commonly used changes frequently. Some practitioners suggest "established" or "consistent" criteria be used instead. Might existing insurance industry practice be used in establishing acceptable cholesterol levels?

Common reports generated on life insurance applicants describe an increase in the decline rates at increasingly worse cholesterol levels relative to the population, as well as link life insurance coverage to preferred best, preferred non-tobacco, standard plus, standard, table 2, table 4, table 6, table 8, and table 10 health classes. The two predominant organizations responsible for annually revising public guidelines on cholesterol management are the American Heart Association and the American College of Cardiology. Organizations with annuity products offer additional guarantees over life insurance contracts and operate portions of business profit at underwriting losses. Individuals with a better cholesterol profile than what is sought may have larger face amounts issued by some companies when several table rated contracts are utilized in a co-insurance arrangement underwriting case. Table rated health classes describe an insured's elevated risk of death. Moreover, it releases a mortality study on hypercholesterolemia using influence from some life office reinsurance treaties sampling up to amounts of up to $60 million for each proposed selected risk. Life contracts profit can vary. The premiums required for one company to issue a $10 million life contract on an applicant with very low cholesterol are possibly lower than the premiums required for another company to issue a $10 million life contract on an applicant with very high cholesterol.

The topic aims to study the cholesterol level at which it is considered acceptable in life insurance assessment. It might consider the insurance industry standards for acceptable cholesterol levels of proposed insured and provide an approach to establishing these thresholds.

3. Factors Influencing Cholesterol Levels and Health Risk Assessment

Due to the relationship between cholesterol and health and their interest in mortality and morbidity risks, life and health insurance companies use the information gained from health risk assessment tools, such as cholesterol, in their underwriting and premium rate setting. Insurers use several models and guidelines such as standard risk classification and/or rating schedules, various manual rates, and commissioned actuarial reports to guide business decisions. However, the vast majority of applicants are still expected to disclose all information that may influence their insurability at the time of application. It is therefore necessary for a life insurance company to be able to understand and interpret an applicant's cholesterol measurements.

Total cholesterol levels among individuals are influenced by several factors such as diet (saturated fats and trans fats), weight, exercise and physical state, age, gender, genetics, and family history, medical conditions (e.g. diabetes (type I and II), thyroid disorders), medications, illicit drug use, and alcohol consumption. With the exception of genetics/family history, the majority of the factors influence lifestyle habits and our physical state, and therefore our potential susceptibility to ill health. Some factors such as age and gender are unmodifiable and will vary between individuals of the same age range. However, cholesterol levels have been found to start rising from as early as seven years of age. Abnormal lipid levels in childhood are a predictive risk factor for heart disease in adulthood. As a result, some life insurance companies have used cholesterol levels as an indicator of adult health risk when assessing the potential insurability of a child.

4. The Relationship Between Cholesterol Levels and Overall Health

Research & Development The insurance company's underwriting guidelines concerning medical conditions and overall mortality rates are largely based on recent data and official releases from the World Health Organization, among other organizations. Most of the findings from these resources are from major populations, comprising millions of people. They include vast amounts of individuals with different cholesterol profiles and different likelihoods of developing health problems. In an effort to minimize the health and mortality risks they take on, insurance companies often verify and supplement the medical record with a laboratory commitment appointment. Such blood tests often focus on validating that an applicant's medical record is accurate; blood pressure, BMI, and cholesterol levels are often checked. Therefore, the so-called assessment of risk that agencies carry out is largely based on examining associations between cardiovascular disease-related conditions and cholesterol levels in insurance candidate populations.

Health implications of cholesterol levels High cholesterol can negatively affect an individual's well-being. It is closely related to developing cardiovascular diseases, which often result from the progress of atherosclerosis, a condition that has to do with excessive plaque accumulation in arteries. In the long run, this can lead to heart attacks, stroke, aortic aneurysm, or peripheral artery disease. Notably, the prevalence of these conditions and their risk is closely tied to cholesterol. There is also ongoing research showing that cholesterol influences non-atherosclerosis-related medical conditions and overall mortality, and that consuming excessive amounts of cholesterol can directly cause harm.

5. Implications of High Cholesterol on Life Insurance Premiums

High Cholesterol example in a term life insurance policy: John is a 33-year-old male who is in great shape. He's 6 feet 1 inch, 183 pounds and his only health concern is his high cholesterol. He's working with his doctor to lower it but the doc is skeptical and says I should also be aware of it. Needless to say, things in John's life are dandy. He doesn't want to put a burden on his family if something were to happen so he's looking to purchase a 20-year term life insurance policy with a death benefit of $1,000,000. He wants to have a rate that is locked in and won't change throughout the term. Because John has no other medical issues, he may potentially be rated with what we would call a flat extra. In layman's terms, this is a premium surcharge on top of the standard rate of insurance costs. This percentage will be much more substantial than the average cholesterol elevator because the chances of him needing to use the policy sooner rather than later.

The significance of having an acceptable or low cholesterol level when talking about insurance is because an insurance company will take great consideration in the amounts of cholesterol in relation to the probability of a claim. For example, high cholesterol represents poor lifestyle choices (a junk food enthusiast, an alcoholic) or underlying illnesses (cancer, diabetes) which could potentially stir the waters. It's possible that the insurance company would deem you uninsurable and not even approve you for a policy. The individual would then be forced to find a high-risk life insurance alternative which costs an arm and a leg. In other scenarios, having high cholesterol could increase the premium of a current policy. Life insurance premium rates are rated/determined by a number of factors including current health conditions. The higher the risk, the higher the cost.

6. Strategies for Lowering Cholesterol Levels

Medication: In the event of dangerously low cholesterol levels and no explanation as to why it is so, the person should refrain from using any of the mentioned interventions without professional medical advice. Individuals with very high cholesterol levels might consider taking a statin, which has been shown to lower cholesterol levels. The United States Preventive Service Task Force published a comprehensive online article on the subject in 2016. As per their findings, adults aged 40 to 75 should be evaluated by their doctor. If they have one of the following four: diabetes, extraction from the highest 10 percent of those examined, cholesterol readings of 130 or greater, or untreated cholesterol totals of 190 or above, the doctor can advise treatment with statins, assuming the clinician agrees. The 2018 study adds more cholesterol information from over 400,000 individuals in the UK, generally conforming to the stance that statins might be valuable for millions more people. When analyzing insurance claims forms submitted by persons with direct-to-consumer prescriptions, a study found that the claims were not processed if patients did not pick up their statin prescriptions. There is, therefore, a chance that clients are not consuming as many medications as they claim.

Lifestyle modifications: Dietary adjustments play a crucial role in the prevention of cholesterol. High consumption of fruits and vegetables, as well as regular physical activity, have been shown to have positive effects. A diet based on whole grains and higher fiber intake has proven to be effective. High fiber intake is associated with low levels of cardiovascular disease. Incorporation of plant sterols can also help; they reduce low-density lipoprotein, a major form of cholesterol transported in the blood. A study including 51 adults with mild to moderately elevated cholesterol levels discovered that adding plant sterols, derived from soybean and pine tree oils, to a typical "Mediterranean" diet resulted in a considerable reduction of cholesterol. Continuing research has validated that patients with high levels of low-density lipoprotein cholesterol can profit from taking plant sterols. Plant sterols would result in a reduction of up to ten percent in a patient's cholesterol level if they consumed at least two grams per day within that eight-week period.

Strategies for managing cholesterol: As already mentioned, there are different interventions available for reducing cholesterol levels.

7. Dietary Interventions and Nutrition for Cholesterol Management

Due to differences in fat and cholesterol within animal products, there was once a recommendation for limiting animal-based proteins. Based on large reviews of the literature, the recommendations were changed to limiting dietary cholesterol to 300mg of cholesterol per day for the general population - this encompasses dietary guidelines for cholesterol management for people with hyperlipidemia. As the body of knowledge expands, the more up-to-date guidelines have loosened the focus on the amount of dietary cholesterol that we get directly from foods. New recommendations now stress the importance of limiting foods that are high in saturated and trans-fat over dietary cholesterol. Overall, the most up-to-date nutritional recommendations for a heart-healthy diet and cholesterol levels include liberal amounts of fruits, vegetables, whole grains, and omega-3 rich fats. These nutritional automated underwriting guidelines set the stage for a treatment plan from the registered dietitian.

Following a heart-healthy eating plan remains a critical component to cholesterol management. This eating plan can consist of various types of dietary choices, and evidence continues to grow regarding the impact of these nutrients on our overall heart health. Dietary fat, in particular, the role of saturated fats and trans fats, were once targeted as an underlying cause for increases in cholesterol levels. Over the years, researchers have discovered that these two fats negatively impact cholesterol levels in the body. Similarly, dietary cholesterol - which once was associated with high LDL - is now understood to only have a minimal impact on overall cholesterol levels. However, these fats are all still considered components that promote inflammation in the body.

Dietary interventions and nutrition

8. Physical Activity and Exercise Recommendations for Cholesterol Control

Participation in regular physical activity is associated with improvements in several risk factors. Aerobic and resistance exercise programs assist in the management of suboptimal lipid profiles and have also been shown to be effective in reducing total cholesterol, LDL cholesterol, triglyceride, and HDL cholesterol. Discretely, evidence shows that weight loss can also have lipid-lowering effects, with a study by Goff et al. finding that reducing weight can lower triglycerides by approximately 1% for every 1% of weight lost. Those who are relatively sedentary initially experience a greater reduction; however, a reduction is also seen in those who are already very active. When combining exercise with weight loss, the reduction effect is additive, with significant improvements observed. This is one reason why experts from various countries and from many different health and fitness associations recommend a minimum of 150 minutes of moderate-intensity or 75 minutes of vigorous-intensity exercise each week combined with muscle-strengthening activities on two or more days a week to achieve additional health benefits.

Cholesterol plays an important role in numerous bodily functions and is a key feature of cell membranes and the protective function of the nerves. However, managing this fatty substance in your blood is necessary to prevent potentially serious heart conditions. While physical activity and exercise can help people control their cholesterol levels, not all exercises offer the same benefits. This section explores the scientific evidence that supports the use of physical activity to control cholesterol levels. It also discusses the practical applications of exercise in the management of cholesterol levels, such as exercise recommendations and the implications for individuals seeking life insurance. This section also provides answers for the chapter reflective questions.

9. Medication and Medical Interventions for High Cholesterol

The only medical procedure to treat high cholesterol that can bring cholesterol levels down into the normal range is apheresis. It is rarely indicated because of its invasiveness. It requires passing a person's blood through a membrane that removes the LDL and then returns the rest of the blood to the person's body. It is only recommended for those with severe hypercholesterolemia. It is also not a cure; cholesterol will go up again and require repeated treatments. Since apheresis is available in only some centers and the cost is high, access to this procedure is even more limited. The patient's symptoms, medical history, and reason for having high cholesterol need to be considered when deciding on which medication to start. Some patients may have a rare genetic disease that causes many other medical problems and are at very high risk for early heart disease. In this case, very low cholesterol levels are often required for effective prevention treatment. Such individuals are also identified by their LDL cholesterol level being very high. Even though low cholesterol levels may increase the risk of side effects, the benefits of treatment usually outweigh the risk of side effects. In the case of one parent being at high risk, then a cholesterol-lowering medication can help decrease the other risk factors.

There are several different classes of cholesterol-lowering medications that have different mechanisms of action. The main classes are statins, PCSK9 inhibitors, bile acid sequestrants, ezetimibe, fibrates, and niacin. There are several others with different mechanisms of action which are in development. The side effect profile varies by class. In some of the earlier generations of medication, fatigue and muscle aches were common adverse effects, particularly at high doses. Dietary and lifestyle modification to lower cholesterol levels tends not to cause low cholesterol levels on its own.

10. Lifestyle Modifications to Improve Cholesterol Profile

• Data show that the relation of modifiable lifestyle factors with lower levels of cholesterol and improved cholesterol profiles extends to our actions or reactions to stress (type A behavior), the cessation of smoking, the control of alcohol consumption, and marijuana. • Bennett, Tadesse-Duguma, and Gourgoulianis found that the mean serum cholesterol of 21 marijuana users was 4.85 mmol/L, while that of 28 demographically matched controls was 5.01 mmol/L. Does the person suffer from a secondary cause of high cholesterol? • Some subclinical and other endocrinological conditions, such as hypothyroidism, Cushing's syndrome, acromegaly, polycystic ovary syndrome, anabolic steroids, or estrogens, can raise serum cholesterol levels. While some rare cases can see generally high levels of cholesterol, e.g., familial dysbetalipoproteinemia. Medicines for the treatment of these conditions are not associated with impaired motor functions, good compliance with treatment regimens, have low morbidity, and improve the lipid profile. They may improve the insurability of some policyholders. • Control of serologic markers such as CRP or LP-PLA-2 (Lipoprotein-associated phospholipase A2) has some cholesterol-lowering effect when compared to statins or fibrates alone, and future research may result in the commercial availability of these drugs. As this line of inquiry is less than 10 years old, the industry currently is not significantly concerned about this line of inquiry.

11. The Role of Genetics in Cholesterol Levels and Health Risks

These new insights will affect the assessment of risk for possible customers. However, genetic information also presents a range of ethical and practical challenges in underwriting. Genetic information may provide a better view of who is at risk following the purchase of an insurance policy. But insurance regulators and authorities are concerned that people will keep information private if it is worthwhile. Research shows that the health implications for individuals are small in most cases, and people have shown poor understanding of the quantitative assessment of the absolute risk of disease.

It is well known that cholesterol levels in the blood are partly determined by genetics. Genetic studies have provided a lot of insight into the heredity of those who have high or low cholesterol levels, as well as insights into the health implications of this. While cholesterol levels have a clear causal relationship with cardiovascular disease, an increase in the level of cholesterol is also associated with reduced risk for other cause-specific deaths. Historically, mortality from atherosclerosis was inversely associated with levels of cholesterol. This is no surprise, as the human body must maintain a certain level of cholesterol, and some genetic conditions may cause high or low levels of cholesterol that are again associated with health risks.

12. Public Health Initiatives and Policies for Cholesterol Awareness

Public health programs have raised awareness of cholesterol and its purported relationship to heart disease. Agencies of the federal government, private non-profit foundations, and many healthcare systems inform the public about the many desirable reasons to lower serum cholesterol levels. Since the late 1960s, most Americans have regularly reported having had their cholesterol measured, and many have reported discussing their cholesterol levels with their physicians. Since 1975, there has been a persistent decline in the prevalence of high cholesterol and mean serum cholesterol levels among Americans. Trends in fat availability data correlate closely with these statistics. Educational initiatives and health-promotion programs have had a measurable effect on both attitudes and behavior. Other cholesterol-related public health and clinical activities, such as an increasing use of cholesterol-lowering drugs and the National Cholesterol Education Program, were also introduced primarily as educational and health-promotion strategies.

Rigorous lifespan analyses of cholesterol could hinge on large, accessible data collection and statistical analysis. It is important to quantify the relationship between LDL cholesterol and cardiovascular disease to improve the accuracy of the assessment of changes in health and in the population's intake of dietary fats. Public health initiatives could recommend or discourage various dietary patterns by pointing to their effect on cholesterol levels and heart attacks. The makers of these recommendations should specify whether they have changed their focus from direct investigations of diet and heart disease.

13. Technological Innovations in Cholesterol Monitoring and Management

In this trying time, telehealth visits are on the rise. Previously, use of technology in health care was in effect. However, because of the pandemic and lockdown, telehealth took off and is expected to continue to grow by 56% annually. With the increased interest and use of technology, there are some challenges that need to be addressed. Privacy, security, and consumer fears need to be addressed. Used in the right way, these wearables, nutrition monitoring systems, and telemedicine platforms should be of use to patient, provider, and insurance companies. There has, however, been some pushback from physicians about the wearable data collection. The possible data overload and then the addition of meeting a patient who may 'update' or 'modify' a device to make it appear as if they are adherent, may be daunting. Being 'always connected' is for some clients a difficult scenario. Some would rather life insurance underwriting stay separate from the technology. Some would still, even though voluntary, be afraid of the loss of privacy or security.

Advancements in technology continue to expand. These advancements provide new ways to help with cholesterol monitoring and management. Many wearable devices track and store cholesterol levels. Telemedicine platforms allow patients to meet with dietitians and receive diet plans, nutrition coaching, and support. Many mobile applications also provide personalized nutrition, meal plans, recipes, and shift access to food purchases and delivery. With the increased use of these wearables and telemedicine platforms, physicians can now access meaningful data or track a patient's activity, nutrition, and lab results. When using a combination of physical activity data, nutrition information, and cholesterol results, the information is more robust in determining if a patient is adhering to recommendations on how to improve their health and lower their cholesterol. Also, voluntary use of these systems is thought to, in general, create a more adherent patient population. Insurance companies are now looking at how these external data sources can be used and if they can be incorporated into the life insurance underwriting process.

14. The Future of Cholesterol Assessment in Life Insurance

The changes and developments in law, science and technology could simplify the assessment of the future of clients/society to some extent and/or change the focus from behaviour/phenotype based underwriting to health/genome-based underwriting. Part of the use of panels has been the discussion if and to what extent panels are predictive for applicants' mortality. Moreover, the requirement of the use of software as well as the technical implementation for the application of a genetic humane underwriting panel are not very different between death and life insurance. In death insurance, artificial intelligence may be allowed to be optimized on the basis of the fact that if an individual should die in the near future it most of the time does not have a too dramatic influence on the prediction and, if the estimated for example the risk of not returning payment of premium is high, information like blood tests could be taken into account in those models, in order not to be competitive in the market for the millions of people. If the risk/premium is too high, one could deny liability without using the results of the examination of a panel with vulnerable genes in the future. This would reduce the danger of adverse selection. In classical life re/practice and products, future complications are relevant and the immediate impact of risk factors (factors like smoking status, weight, serum level of biomarkers, ... and medical history). Health insurance applicants frequently wish to know if insurance cover is available. An insurance giving a large degree of personalisation will generally attract a low risk profile, as only applicants who expect a large benefit find the insurance cover attractive. For this, a minimal risk rating could be necessary. A larger number of insurers are expected to become interested in selling health insurance products using large levels of personalisation. More personalized health and life cover would lead to larger demand, competition and increased availability in personalized policies such as this. This might lead to increased competition among insurers such that the increase in expected cost for an insurer who starts offering a $p = 1/2g$ cover is greater than $p(K2 - K1 + K2)$ and consequently exactly $p(1 - p)(K2 - K1)(1 - g)$ policies would be acquired on $p = xf$ displayed in equation (2b).

The major regulatory change that could have a potential impact on cholesterol assessment in the coming years is related to big data and its ethical, clinical, and insurance-related implications. Here, two main changes in the development of technology were identified, i.e., growing possibilities in biobanking and the possibilities of metabolomics and proteomics to exert precise medicine. As an example, it could have a potential impact on developments in science, but for insurance purposes less targeted diagnostics would be developed, because for insurance purposes generally a rough distinction between groups and not the unfavourable ones in a group is relevant. Regulation aimed at ensuring the protection of individuals will continue in time and was focused on the

GDPR, which is relevant, since some insurers criticize the limit for the use of biomarkers in life insurance. It remains to be seen if, in the future, insurers will still be allowed to request or analyse blood tests for health insurance purposes without ethical restrictions, or, be allowed to apply the right not to know of individuals, as expressed in the GDPR and NHLGS.

15. Conclusion and Key Takeaways

In order to mitigate the effects of that on disease-related costs, it may encourage pre-adverse selection by high-cholesterol applicants. A fresh wave of cholesterol medications, applicants influenced or not, because they may choose to inform themselves and engage in a suitable program of lifestyle, medication, or therapy. In an era where health education is soaring and e-patients want to manage their health more, the most likely long-term impact would be a better-educated population with growing knowledge to use. Lifestyle, genetics, and prescription policy all have an effect on lowering difficult-to-treat cholesterol levels. This essay provides a cogent argument for the importance of cholesterol. A understanding of cholesterol is important but only the first step.

Cholesterol plays a significant role in the assessment of heart disease, healthcare, and life insurance. It requires appropriate management on the part of insurance companies, healthcare providers, and patients to achieve the best outcome. "Good cholesterol" traps bad cholesterol in the arteries at such low levels that they can be picked up by the liver and discarded easily. Anybody with a level of low LDL above 160 should edit his or her diet and speak to the doctor accordingly. In terms of HDL, values above 35 are regarded as healthy, but they offer more protective effects as they increase. Although this method has been discovered to be a good complement, there are some worries that it raises the chances of false positives.